# LIVING YOUR LIFE IN REVERSE

---

## LUCY RUTH

# CONTENTS

*Introduction*   vii
1. Living In Reverse   1
2. Sun Facts   7
3. Reset   10
4. Sugar   13
5. Food For Thought   19
6. Salts   23
7. Fats   28
8. Vitamins   36
   Who is Lucy Ruth?   47

Copyright © Lucy Ruth, 2020

Publisher's Note

This book was printed and bound in Canada. All rights reserved.

All rights reserved. No part of this book may be reproduced or transmitted in any form or by any means, electronic or mechanical, including photocopying, recording, or by any information storage and retrieval system except by a review who may quote brief passages in a review to be printed in a magazine, newspaper, or on the Web without permission in writing from Lucy Ruth.

Although the author and publisher have made every effort to ensure the accuracy and completeness of the information contained in this book, we assume no responsibility for errors, inaccuracies, omissions, or any inconsistency herein. The advice and strategies contained herein may not be suitable for your situation. You should consult with a professional where appropriate. Neither the publisher nor the author shall be liable for damages arising.

*I dedicate this book to God, who gave me the wisdom to write and empower others. To my mom in heaven, I never had the chance to say goodbye, and I will always love, to my family, friends, and networks. I love you all.*

# INTRODUCTION

**Writing my first book**

*Debunk & Develop Your Mind* has opened my eyes and made me passionate about writing more books in order to help others improve their lifestyles by making small life changes. This book will help you change the way you look at foods and help you develop new ideas into healthy living by going back to the old ways of life.

Now, I did not plan to write this book. God dropped it into my spirit, and I loved the idea and wanted to share it. I woke up one Sunday morning, and as usual, I went to have a shower. While taking a shower, my mind began to wander, and I slipped into a relaxed mode. I love it when this happens. When I'm in a relaxed mode, I find myself singing, praying, and sometimes even crying. As I am writing this book, I have reminisced how many times I have had showers to cool me down or just let the shower and the natural undiluted no preservative lubricant of tears work together in releasing those endorphins and let go of some bad days.

Now, this special shower opened my eyes about how one can actually live a life in reverse and live a healthy lifestyle; YES U GOT THAT RIGHT! LIVE A REVERSED LIFE.

So how does one live a reversed life and live healthily? The following pages are going to inform you of how you can revert back to the lifestyle that we are intended to live. I'll share with you some natural ways that you can tap into the universe and heal yourself using resources found in the earth. We're headed to a time where it's important to live abundantly in all areas of our lives. To do that, you'll need the right tools and resources.

I am going to share journeys from all walks of life that have helped many people live long, healthy lifestyles without relying on a lot of medication.

In ancient times families spent time with their families playing games instead of watching TV. There's nothing wrong with watching TV but obsessively watching hockey, baseball, basketball, soccer, and many more every weekend, and not taking the time to spend with your families is an unhealthy way of living. A healthier approach is to find time and activities to do with friends and family. Doing this gives you a balanced approach, and you can still watch your sports/TV shows later.

A few weeks ago, I read an article that said, don't be closer to your friends on social media and lose the ones you are sitting next to. This is so true. Our generation is now obsessed with our friends' next door instead of my immediate circle of friends.

Our generation is filled with pride, and we don't love one another, why do I say that? I have seen and witnessed parents that don't allow their kids to play with their neighbor's kids. We need to put a STOP to this behavior as we are not doing our kids any good. Most childhood memories involve playing dodgeball and hopscotch with my friends from my street. As parents, let's take a step back and reflect and be role models for our kids.

I get it. You might not like the guy or girl next door, but that's you and not your child's choice. Some people can't even stand their own neighbors for reasons unknown. We need to go back to basics and unite our communities.

Let's REVERSE back to the old days where family values were

what brought our societies closer, and our relationships were a bit more intimate.

In modern-day society, I have heard people say, "Oh, I don't talk to my mother or father." I am not here to judge anyone, but what sin has your parent did that is worth unforgiveness?

We all make mistakes, and we all need love, and even those who have committed a crime, the judge gives them a pardon at some point. Rejection from a child or a parent hurts. Why don't we mend our relationships?

Let's reverse our thinking into old times, where they taught us forgiveness and forgive one another more often. There's more unhappiness and resentment in unforgiveness, and in the end, it tends to hurt us more. Forgiveness brings some form of healing. As a result of losing my mother at a young age I have lived the pain and I encourage you to forgive. Try it, and if it doesn't work you, can put it in the to-do list or one of your New Year's resolutions.

My goal is to teach you how to create and live a reversed life so that you can be happier and healthier. You can also utilize the exercises throughout this book to help you jumpstart your new life.

# 1

## LIVING IN REVERSE

―◦―

Growing up in Africa taught me that one doesn't need most of the things that Western life has taught us. For centuries, being in the West has been about materialism. You often hear people saying; I want a house, I want a car, I want new clothes and I want more money. While this is not bad, we have become enslaved to materialism and have lost touch with real life. The side of life that allows us to enjoy the simple things. Things like reading books from the library, breathing clean air, walking to our destinations.

Most people are all about them. Rarely do you find people to ask you, "How are you doing?" And actually wait for a response. Seldom do you see people enjoying a walk in the park or having small talk after work? It's more common to see people constantly on the go. Snapping pictures of their location, taking videos of their experiences, posing with their latest gadget or article of clothing. Human beings have lost their personal touch, and it shows.

The love of materialism and not being content with what we have has led our generation into some depression, anxiety, and debt. So many people had become consumed with cars, vacations, houses, flashy clothes that when the ride was over it, left them feeling empty.

People forgot how great it was just to have the essentials of life at the tip of your fingers. We lost track of the importance of life.

We need to reverse and go back to the basics where family, food, shelter, and clothing is enough. We need to revisit the time when money, social media likes, and popularity wasn't a priority. I yearn for the days where we eat dinner and attend parties to enjoy the conversation. I miss the moments that we enjoyed the camaraderie. I appreciated having stability; now, some view stability as boring. When did we get to this point? Does everything have to be about what we have, where we live, or what we drive?

Growing up, having family dinners consisted of talking, laughing, and sharing stories. Now, every dinner, party, or gathering includes posing for pictures and selfies. Is this really what we are concerned about when our environment is shifting right before our eyes?

I long for the times when life had substance. We've become a shallow group of people. Instead of dreaming and anticipating the good, we demand it. We chase after it. Now, we live in a constant state of wanting and because of the love for the things we want, we cause all sorts of chaos in the world. Our desires become so ingrained in us that we chase it down. And when we finally get it, we're still unsatisfied. We have to go out and get more; we become greedy. And greed destroys people.

Our greed doesn't only destroy people, but we are also damaging our environment due to excessive waste and overproducing of stuff that we already have. We now live in a society where we compete and instead of partnering together. When this happens, we waste our time, money, and resources. We become greedy, selfish even.

Have you ever stopped to think, why does the world need 5,500 airlines? This doesn't include the individual number of fleets each airline holds. One popular airline has a fleet size of 1,789. There is an estimate of 39,000 in the world. Why don't investors partner up and buy existing shares into companies that are already operating to reduce our carbon footprint? Why are we so bent on having our own rather than building together?

Our access to luxury and privilege has made us lazy. Instead of us using our limbs to move about, we depend on devices. Thanks to technology, we don't even have to think for ourselves anymore thanks to Smartphones. We are driving our kids to schools when we live so close to the school that we can walk them there. We can do so much for the environment if we just walked more!

And what's wrong with walking? How do you think our ancestors got around before there were cars? Exactly. We should consider this before we hop in our cars for a five-minute drive that could cause more harm to our environment, and ultimately us, the people.

I believe it's time for us to get back in the swing of things. It's time for people to get in alignment with the natural state this world should be in. I believe the catastrophe and calamity we're facing is a sign that we need to go back to our way of living when life was simple. All we need to do is reverse our steps and get back to our rightful places. We have to honor our environment so that we can survive.

If we reverse a few steps back, we can change and save the environment for future generations. If we keep moving at this pace, the environment will be forever changed. It's our responsibility to honor and protect the land. And so far, we've failed. However, it's not too late for us to turn things around. This pandemic that we're facing is not a coincidence. It's a sign that we need to come together, regroup, and revert to a time when life was good. But first, we have to take action. And massive action at that. We need to reverse our lifestyles to save the planet from greenhouse gases.

## What Are Greenhouse Gases?

GREENHOUSE GASES ARE gas molecules that have the property of absorbing infrared radiation (net heat energy) emitted from Earth's surface and reradiating it back to Earth's surface, thus contributing to the phenomenon known as the greenhouse effect. Carbon dioxide, methane, and water vapor are the most important greenhouse gases, and they have a profound effect on the energy budget of the Earth system despite making up only a fraction of all atmospheric gases. Concentrations of greenhouse gases have varied substantially during Earth's history, and these variations have driven substantial climate changes at a wide range of timescales (source Encyclopedia Britannica).

What I'm trying to say is that we're messing up our planet, and here's how. When using gasses such as Carbon dioxide, methane, and nitrous oxide in our day to day activities, we're contributing to the unbalance of the earth's atmosphere. And when the atmosphere is unbalanced, it affects not only the ecosystem but all of us – the economy and communities, too.

So, what are some ways you can avoid using greenhouse gases? Glad you asked! Here are a few ways you can help reverse the earth:

- Start using energy-efficient light bulbs
- Exchange your gas stove for an electric stove
- When you're not using your computers, TVs and any other electronics – unplug them
- Use a heat pump instead of a furnace
- If it's possible, take public transit or ride with others
- Stop reading for a second, look around you and see how many plugged appliances are wasting energy while lying idle. Unplug them and save energy.

I KNOW it can take some getting used to, but taking a step-in reverse will be a great thing for the people and this planet.

## Long Live the People

GROWING UP IN ZIMBABWE, I never saw any of my grandparents take painkillers as often as we do in the Western world. I have witnessed and seen people live to be 100 years old in poverty without a lot of healthcare. Some of them even tilled fields up to 75 years of age. It was very common to see healthy men and women 75 years or more. Eating healthy foods is a way of life for them, which is why so many people in the older generation are still doing well. The Western older generation has a different experience.

All they have ever known is how to make your own food, can it, and store it using natural methods. In third world countries in rural areas, most people don't have access to electricity, clean water, fridges, and freezers. Guess what? That doesn't affect their quality of life.

They don't have bills, bills, bills, and more bills. They drink water out of wells, and they eat organic foods. Their foods are organic because they cultivate, grow, and harvest the foods themselves without the use of pesticides. They have free-range eggs and chickens.

So why don't they have body pains as compared to us here in the first world? How can someone without clean water live a long life?

According to life in the Western world, you won't be able to survive without Spring or Distilled water. And you can't forget the lemon! It's unheard of for people in the Western world to keep their meat out of the freezer. They wouldn't know what to do if their food is not stored in a refrigerator.

While there are some health-conscious people on the Western side of the world, most are only eating organic fruits and vegetables because it's trendy. And they're certainly not working up to the age of 75 because they have to retire! Retire and do nothing all day.

Life doesn't have to be chaotic, stressful, financially burdensome, or unhealthy. There is a way to live a life free of financial and societal pressure. Want to know the secret?

### Here Is The Secret

With all the health products on the market right now, it may seem as if there's some magic pill or drink to help you live past 75 years old.

While there is no pill or drink, there is one secret to a long and healthy life.

The secret is in their day to day activities. Yep, the secret is to be active! There are three keys to why people in third-world countries live less chronic lifestyles than those in Western Civilization.

1. They are in the fields and gardens when it's planting or harvesting seasons. Participating in the process of growing foods keeps people energetic. It's also a good way to exercise.
2. Their foods are organic, and they don't eat a lot of canned and processed foods like us. Because third-world country citizens do not have access to grocery stores, restaurants, and fast-food drive-thru windows, they eat healthier foods.
3. Their diets contain a lot of whole grains. Since eating whole grains such as wheat, rice, and oats, they have a lower chance of getting several diseases.

Now, don't get me wrong, they do get ill, but not at the rate that we get ill. It is rarely as severe, since their immune system is more healthy. That being said, they do have an advantage due to the hot climate. The weather is mostly hotter than ours, so they have more access to sunny days, which gives them more vitamin D. Since we're on the topic of the sun, let's talk about how important it is for us to get a little sun in our lives on a consistent basis.

## 2

## SUN FACTS

―⁂―

The sun has such an important role in life. It literally gives things life. It plays a pretty major role in the circle of life. According to many researchers, the sun plays an important role in our overall health. Spending a little time each day exposed to the sun helps you sleep better, have a great attitude, get stronger bones, and even a better immune system.

Think about it for a minute; why are there less people with the flu in the summer? The answer is the sun has an ability to kill certain bacteria and some viruses. We use heat to kill bacteria in our foods, so my logical thinking is, the heat kills some of the airborne viruses, thus keeping people in warmer regions somewhat healthier.

So what is it about the sun that it helps us be healthier? The sun produces vitamin D, which is of major importance to our overall health.

My own observations of the sun are that it brings so much happiness to people. We all hear cars driving by playing loud music during the summer months. The days spent at the beach are so relaxing. The soothing sound of the waves of the sea is the perfect soundtrack to enjoy the sun; the birds chirp louder, the air brings so much peace and tranquility. Some who are blessed enough to have cottages by the beach enjoy summer sunsets, and it brings life to a whole new meaning. There's less stress with the sun warming up the earth.

Although there are some healthy reasons to intake the sun, there are also some unhealthy reasons not to get too much sun. While the warmth of the sun can encourage you to stay in it for long periods of time, you'll need to monitor just how long you spend in the sun. If you overexpose yourself, you can likely have skin damage. Try and avoid excessive sunburns and suntans whilst you are enjoying the sun. Along with vitamin D, the sun also distributes UV Rays. That being said, depending on your geographical location, it is important to educate yourself about the UV rays.

UV (Ultraviolet) radiation has effects both beneficial and harmful to human health, so be careful and take it easy with the sun. Though it's fun being in the sun, it has some risks involved with it.

When you're outdoors enjoying the sun, always find shade, wear sunscreen, and cover up with light summer clothing that is breathable. It is recommended that one protects themselves from the UV rays from 11 AM to 3 PM because the UV index is higher. It is recommended that you apply the same principle on both sunny and cloudy days since the sun's rays can get through light clouds, mist, and fog.

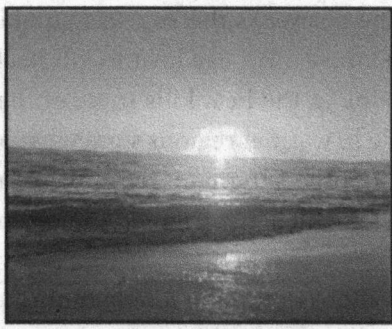

THE BEST TIME TO enjoy the sun is at sunset. I took this picture from Carpinteria, California. I must admit there's a peacefulness that comes from watching the sunset.

Make time to see and watch a few sunsets by the beach in the summer. I know firsthand how relaxing it can be, but I have heard some people say it also helps with depression. Follow closely on Social Media, and you will see that many people love to take shots of sunsets all over the world. It's a great way to reset and retreat from the day.

Reconnect with nature and take time to relax and rejuvenate your mind. It will help the process of living life in reverse. Be intentional and make time to do this. One way is to set a schedule to remind you to connect regularly.

| Sunday | Monday | Tuesday | Wednesday | Thursday | Friday | Saturday |
|--------|--------|---------|-----------|----------|--------|----------|
|        |        |         |           |          |        |          |
|        |        |         |           |          |        |          |
|        |        |         |           |          |        |          |

**Benefits of Vitamin D**

SO NOW THAT we're clear on the benefits of the sun, receiving vitamin D, let's talk about the benefits this particular vitamin brings.

Vitamin D has many nutritional benefits for men, women, and children. Vitamin D plays a key role in the proper absorption of calcium for strong bones and teeth and has been shown to support colon, breast, prostate, ovarian, heart, and colorectal health.

The sun isn't the only way to intake this important vitamin; you can also access vitamin D through tuna, salmon, orange juice, dairy products, and some cereals. Make sure to include this vitamin in your diet, preferably via the sun.

Write a journal of how much sun exposure you get throughout the year and keep track of the times and how often.

## 3
# RESET

―⚮―

The state of the world that we're in is scary for some, and a new start for others. I can allow the opinions of others to persuade my thoughts about the pandemic, but the truth is, I think what's happening is a sign that we need to simply start over. We need to reset.

Reset? Yes! Let's reset and go back to the old ways of living where families played board games and spent quality time together. Let's reset and limit the number of times we play video games online; let's replace it by human interactions. Let's have dinner without looking down at our phones the entire time. Let's just enjoy the present moment with our fellow mankind. It may not seem like it, but by doing this, we will save the environment.

Reducing the time we spend on our phones leads us one step closer to living a life in reverse. Before regular phones became Smartphones, we made more time to spend with our loved ones. We enjoyed the fundamental joys of life. How can we get back to that place in life? By doing a mental reset.

We can do a mental reset and reduce screen time by reading more books. Our eyes are probably begging to be free from staring at screens all day. Mobile devices are very convenient, but not very healthy for long term usage. I attended a seminar about eye health, and it is believed that by 2050 half the world will be myopic. Everyone will be walking with their phones glued to their face just to read a text or dial a number. Unfortunately, most people will be suffering from eye growth and will require surgery.

Why is this our fate? Well, it's because our lifestyles are being spent more indoors than outdoors. We're binge-watching Netflix, scrolling on our phones, and sitting in front of our computers. Our current lifestyles are unhealthy.

The lack of people having an outdoor life and our addictions to Gadgets is a big part of why our generation has some of these chronic ailments. Our lifestyle choices keep us so far from the lifestyle our ancestors experienced, giving us a different quality and perspective on life.

Although the older generation didn't have advanced health systems, their lives were free from chronic ailments. It wasn't common for so many young people to have cancer or the other diseases our bodies have been attacked by. The only way for our generation is to make some changes. We must act in order to save ourselves.

*SEE ARTICLE BELOW, *written by Linda Carroll who is a health contributor to NBC.*

THERE WAS a research that was done, and the researchers analyzed data from a central database of state cancer registries, focusing on new diagnoses of 30 types of cancer, 12 of which are associated with excess weight, from 1995 to 2014. They had complete data from 25 states that represent about two-thirds of the U.S. population.

In that 20-year period, there were about 14.7 million new cases of the 30 cancers. For at least eight cancers, including smoking-related and HIV-associated cancers, the incidence rates dropped.

But for six of the 12 obesity-related cancers — colorectal, endometrial, gallbladder, kidney, pancreas, and multiple myeloma — there was a steady increase in incidence over the years, with larger increases in younger adults.

The annual rise in new cases of kidney cancer, for example, was 6.23 percent among people aged 25-29, but about 3 percent in the 45-49 age group. Similarly, pancreatic cancer incidence rose 4.3 percent each year for 25- to 29-year-olds but less than 1 percent annually among people aged 45-49.

Overall, rates of colorectal, endometrial, pancreatic and gallbladder cancers in millennials — young adults born around 1985 — were about double the rates seen in people born in the 1950s at the same age, the researchers note.

*DISCLAIMER: I am not guaranteeing that one doesn't get cancer by reversing our lifestyles. I am just raising awareness in order for our generation to take positive action.*

# 4

# SUGAR

One of the ways we can start reversing our lives is to change our eating habits. The first habit we need to change is our sugar intake. True enough, sugar is delicious. Unfortunately, too much sugar can be very unhealthy for us. When we have too much sugar in our diet, it leads to weight gain, acne, depression, diabetes, and cavities. I was surprised at the research I found out just how many people get cavities from sugar. Studies show that over 90% of people in Western civilization will have some type of tooth decay related to their sugar intake. This is not the case in other parts of the world.

The reason why people in developing countries don't have as many cavities is their diet. It doesn't contain a lot of sugar. Unlike here in the Western part of the world, our society starts at a very young age to indulge in bad sugars. The younger we get exposed to unhealthy eating habits, the harder it is to cure the issue. And when it comes to having too much sugar, we have to get our teeth checked regularly. That means we have to go to the dentist. And we all know how people feel about the dentist.

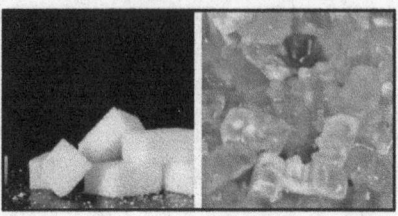

Most kids don't enjoy dental visits because let's face it, they're not fun. However, having healthy teeth is very important and we have to learn what are the proper things to eat and what should be avoided to maintain healthy teeth. As a parent, one is forced to do what's right by taking them for preventative cleanings and care. My daughter is terrified of the dentist, and I hate fillings, yet I LOVE CANDY, and so do my kids. Because of this, I make sure that we get our teeth taken care of regularly.

Today's generation is overindulging in processed sugars because it's always advertised to us. It's even offered as a gift! Think about it. Almost every season 365 days a year our kids are eating candy. Christmas let's stock our stockings with candy. Valentine's day at school has more candy, Easter more candy, and the mother of all sugars is Halloween.

Now, don't get me wrong I enjoy every one of these seasons just like everyone else, but at what point do we say, *I think we have indulged in enough sugar for the year.* And let's face it, we won't say it often. Why? Because sugar is delicious! However, that doesn't mean we must overindulge.

You're probably thinking out loud, "Do we overindulge?" The answer is yes, yes, we do. Let us not forget, that in between these events we are eating cakes and drinking juices loaded with sugar, and if you love coffee with sugar as I do, then you're indulging in even more sugar. As if sugar isn't enough, when you add caffeine, it's really bad! Nowadays some people can't function without energy drinks.

And we all know that diet coke doesn't taste the same as the original coke. Why? Because of less sugar.

So what do we do? Get an original coke because we need our sugar fix.

As for me, it's sugar all the way! I love fizzy drinks and their sugars. No reduced sugar in my drinks. I admit that this is one of the things I'll be working on as I shift into living life in the reverse. And I hope that after you read this chapter, that you do the same.

Why do we continue to consume sugar the way we do, and we know it's no good for us? The answer is simple, our generation suffers from a sugar addiction, and the reason why nobody says anything is because sugar is a 77.5-billion-dollar industry.

Yep, you read that right!

Having my own addiction to sugar, I decided to learn more about what it is I'm so infatuated with. Here are some interesting facts I found about sugar.

The sugar industry subsumes the production, processing, and marketing of sugars (mostly saccharose and fructose). Globally, most sugar is extracted from sugar cane (~80 % predominantly in the tropics) and sugar beet (~ 20%, mostly in temperate climates like in the U.S. or Europe).

Sugar is used in our favorite soft drinks, sweetened beverages, convenience foods, fast food, candy, confectionery, baked products, and other sweetened foods.

Sugar subsidies have driven market costs for sugar well below the cost of production. As of 2018, 3/4 of world sugar production was not traded on the open market. The global market for sugar and sweeteners was some $77.5 billion in 2012, with sugar comprising an almost 85% share, growing at a compound annual growth rate of 4.6%.

Globally in 2018, around 185 million tons of sugar was produced, led by India with 35.9 million tons, followed by Brazil and Thailand. There are more than 123 sugar-producing countries, but only 30% of the produce is traded on the international mark (source Wikipedia).

## Can We Let Sugar Go?

AFTER ALL THAT I know about sugar, it should be easy to just let it go, right? Wrong! It's hard breaking habits, especially habits as good as sugar.

What makes letting go of sugar so hard is that it's everywhere; left, right, and center everywhere you look sugar is present. And it's pretty hard to hide from it. Why, why, why is it hard to let go of you, mother sugar? We need to stop our addiction! That's the only way we'll get back to living life the right way.

As I mentioned earlier in third world countries where sugar consumption is not as high, you find that disease is not as rampant. Why are cancer rates high in the developed world? The answer in my own thinking is the diet. We are eating too many sugars, salts, fats, and too many preservatives. That, combined with our sedentary lives, is the reason why we are faced with a world full of chronic health problems.

## Health Is Everything

THE OLDER GENERATION enlightened us about the importance of our health. If you ask older people, they will tell you what their diets consisted of, simply because they want you to be healthy, too. I just love older people! They are old because they did something right. Despite what others think, getting older is a gift, a beautiful process that I'm looking forward to. Connecting with older people is a great way to start living life in reverse. You'll learn a thing or two that will help you.

Talking to older people will give you some insight on how to naturally improve your health. They know remedies that are not found in Western medicine. Plus, they have great stories! Make time to connect with the elders in your family, such as grandparents, great uncles, and aunts. If you're grandparents, aunts or uncles aren't around anymore; I suggest volunteering in nursing homes where you see and hear what other old people did in their lifetimes. It will open your eyes, deepen your experience, and increase your wisdom.

In my experiences with the older generation, I noticed that they paid more attention to the foods they consumed. They ate a lot more organic foods than we do. They cooked more foods from scratch than we do nowadays. And because of this, they tend to have lived much longer lives.

### Food Shopping in the 21st Century

I GET IT, times have changed, and to my surprise, while walking down the grocery aisle in the frozen foods department, I saw that they now sell frozen French toast. Can you believe that? *Frozen French toast!* Common millennials, I have to know, what are we doing with our time that we can't make fresh French toast?

Cooking food as I knew it growing up drastically changed. We've gotten more comfortable with others preparing our food than cooking our own. We've put our trust in others, and now we really don't know what we're eating. Frankly put, we've gotten lazy in the kitchen.

I understand the world we live in is so busy we don't even have time to cook fresh meals because we have to work and as well raise kids with our demanding lifestyles. After work, one might find themselves so tired that one has to just sit and watch their favorite TV shows, or we have to spend an hour on social media (just my sense of humor).

Come on, guys! We can do this. We can cook our own food. We can make the time to cook fresh food from scratch. We are more than capable of providing our families with healthy meals. I say let's do this together. Let's put a plan of action together and make this happen. Are you with me?

### Buy In Bulk

My grandma's generation didn't spend every week in grocery stores. They didn't have time; also, they bought food in bulk, so they had no reason to go back and forth to the grocery store. That particular lifestyle made them save food because they only cooked what they bought.

Our generation wastes a lot of food. This is because we eat based on our desires, not what we have. We need to learn to be minimalist with food by eating whole foods, which makes us full for longer periods.

On your marks, Get set, ready, and **GO!**
Let's **REVERSE OUR LIFESTYLES!**

## 5

# FOOD FOR THOUGHT

In ancient times people used to farm and grow their own foods. People came together to ensure the town had food for everyone to eat. If more farms existed, we'd have cheaper foods, and we'd be able to afford organic foods in order to live healthier longer lives. Nowadays we barely have people who want to work at the farms, so that means we're importing more food thereby making the price of food expensive and that results in us being forced to eat what our pockets can afford.

Farmers can't run the farm alone. They need the townspeople. Because locals are not interested in farm work, this makes it hard for farmers to produce fresh food and for people to eat healthy food. They rely on foreign workers to be able to provide food for us.

After thinking about this fact, I began to wonder why people aren't interested in doing honest work that not only helps the local community to thrive, but to stay alive. It's because our society has enabled laziness. We've adopted a new way to receive food, so no one wants to help get food the right way. People are now getting too lazy to contribute to society, so no one wants to work on the farm. Unfortunately, people don't see the value in being a farmer. It's a good job! But some people don't see farming that way and miss out on a great opportunity. Let's encourage our future generation to fall in love with agriculture and horticulture. The world's population is growing, so we must prepare and encourage our future leaders about the benefits of having food grown locally. Farming is a recession-proof industry, and depending on what the farmer farms, some farming families earn over a million dollars a year.

## Contributing to Society

ANOTHER THING the older generation did was contribute to society. It was rare for people not to work and embrace being unemployed willingly. It's been socially acceptable to live off of other people. The impact of not having a job doesn't affect some people who are reliant on social welfare. Not contributing to society puts extra stress on those who are. And when people are stressed, it affects other areas of our livelihood as well.

Taking the financial burden of other people is unfair in so many ways. I'd love to stand on my soapbox and share my opinion on this matter, but it won't change anything, anytime soon. Why? Well for starters, the government will pay their rent and provide them food. A good way to continue feeding people who don't have a job is to recommend they work for their food on the farm. This will do two things: help the farmers by contributing and feed your family with integrity. A good example to learn from this, with Coronavirus and travel restrictions, our farmers who rely on foreign workers can't cope at a critical time like this, this means we are going to rely on imported foods.

I know that the grocery stores are more convenient, and you're not used to shopping on a farm, but I want to encourage you to think about doing that. Support your local farmers and buy from them. And if you really want to appreciate fresh foods– start your own garden.

In Brantford, where I live, they have a program for community gardening, which runs from May to October. This is a good way of growing your own foods and eating healthy for a season. I have planted tomatoes, carrots, cucumbers, and lettuce. This is also fun for families with young children. My kids love going to the garden in the summer to water the garden. They enjoy being a part of the food growing process for the foods they later eat. While gardening is great for eating better, it's also very therapeutic.

Asking you to support a farm is so that you can not only support your local community but to also encourage you to eat healthily. And of course, that's not the only way to get fresh fruits and veggies. Another way of eating healthy is by getting to know your city's farmers market.

The farmers market is a local sales event that allows farmers to sell their products directly to consumers instead of wholesalers like grocery stores. Visiting your local farmers market helps you to contribute to your community, get some healthy food, and enjoy a little sun. All things encouraged to help you start living life in reverse.

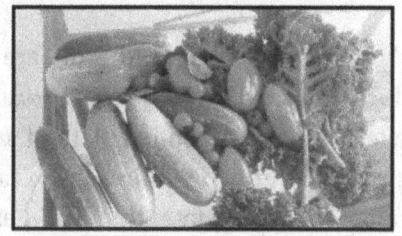

THIS WAS one of my harvests from my community garden. I spent all summer eating fresh cucumbers, tomatoes, and kale. (Find out from your local city councils and get your own and grow your food.) Gardening is also very therapeutic in my experience.

**Farmers Markets**

I talked a little about farmer's markets in the previous chapter, but let's go a little deeper. Now, as I mentioned, farmers markets allow locals to buy food directly from the farmer's, and I love this! They tend to sell fresher food which is healthier because it hasn't gone through a processing plant.

I find my local farmers market to have a good deal on eggs, I buy a crate for $9.00, and that lasts me all month. It's cheaper than buying a dozen for $3.00. I also love that I can get seasonal fruits and veggies that aren't normally stocked in grocery stores. And what about the local jams and jellies? They go so good on fresh biscuits!

I recommend for you to check your city's listing of your local farmers and pay them a visit. This habit is an old habit, but you will eat less processed foods, and you can refill your fresh vegetables and meats on a weekly basis. This is a reversed way of living, which is healthy. Remember, when you buy from farmer's markets, you are also serving the environment from unnecessary food packaging.

## Where Do They Get Their Produce?

IDEALLY, FARMERS' market produce, and fruit are normally grown within a geographical region that is deemed local by the market's management. The term "local" is defined by the farmers' market and usually represents products grown within a given radius measured in miles. Many farmers' markets state that they are producer-only markets and that their vendors grow all products sold. Some farmers' markets do not use the term "producer-only" and may allow resellers of produce, fruit, and other food products.

Some farmers' markets allow vendors to resell vegetables and fruits if they are not available locally due to the time of the year. Vegetables, fruit, meat, and other products resold at farmers' markets are available to vendors through food distributors.

This is a common practice and provides consumers with produce and fruit that are unavailable at certain times of the year. In many markets, resell items are a permanent part of the vendor's inventory. (Wikipedia)

# 6

# SALTS

Okay, so let's talk about salt! I have a love/hate relationship with this seasoning. It tastes oh so good but can be oh so bad. There are many facts about the concerns of salt, yet no matter how negative the facts are, people continue to consume this seasoning at high levels.

So, what exactly is salt? Salt is a mineral compound of sodium chloride. In its natural form as a crystalline mineral, it's known as rock salt. It is found in seawater. Research shows that there are roughly about 35 grams of salt solids per liter of seawater.

According to the government of Canada, Canadians eat roughly 3400 mg of sodium each day, which is double the daily required amount. Who needs that much salt? Furthermore, why are people using this much? This is insane people! Why is it insane?

Too much sodium in our diet may open a can of worms to things like heart disease, stroke, high blood pressure, and many more. Yes, salt makes food taste a little better. Okay, it helps food taste a LOT better. However, it's not necessarily the best way to season our food. While salt is a great addition to a dish, we have to be mindful of the quantity we're consuming. It's best to find other ways to give our foods that salty flavor in a more healthy way. Let's implement changes to our diets and the way we look at certain foods.

Can you imagine your diet without a certain amount of salt? Salt in the right amounts is good for our health. However, due to most foods being mass-produced, it is used for preserving foods, not just adding flavor. The problem with this is that our dependence on eating too many readymade foods increases our salt intake. It's not a wise decision to consume an ingredient that affects our health in such a negative way.

In order to live a reversed lifestyle, you have to cut down on eating lots of readymade foods, so that you can eat fresh home-cooked foods. It's not hard to reduce the amount of salt you're eating. You can definitely control the amount of salt you are consuming. How? Well, by being intentional.

For example, I am a lover of salted popcorn but sometimes I am just too tired to make the popcorn, so ready-made popcorn is the option here. Since ready-made popcorn has way more salt than I need, I now make sure that I have homemade popcorn available for snacking on the weekends.

Now, making popcorn from scratch may seem like a lot of work, but it's not. I use a tablespoon of coconut oil and a few kernels. I swear by coconut oil instead of vegetable oil for this, it just makes the popcorn taste good. I pop the popcorn, and after it's done, I lightly season it with salt—one of my favorite snacks. Feel free to try this method.

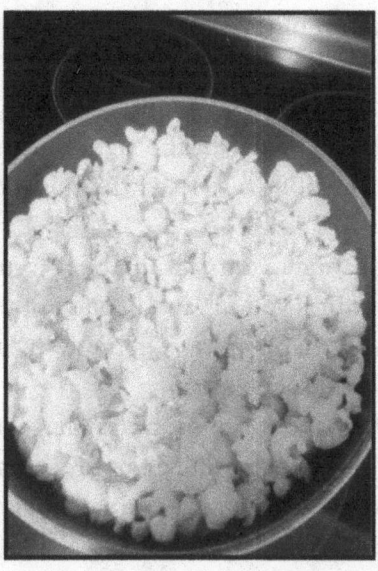

### Other Purposes for Salt

In my rural home of Chivhu in Zimbabwe, my grandma didn't have a freezer, but she often bought beef in bulk. Since she couldn't keep the meat fresh using ice, she learned a different method: salt. Yep, salt played a very important role in keeping my grandma's beef fresh. She would bring the meat home, then dry it seasoned with salt so that flies couldn't lay eggs or germs. The meat will then dry and will be dry stored in a container. And every time she wants beef, she will grab it from the container and boil it then make beef stew. This method helped my grandma preserve food naturally. Now that's a good way of food preservation vs. chemicals.

### Watch That Salt!

IT'S ALMOST impossible to have a good dish without a little sprinkle of salt. I don't know what it is, but it's something about the flavor of this ingredient that just elevates the taste of any food that it compliments.

We have to be mindful of the amount we use so that we don't affect our health.

Let's reverse our diets and reduce sodium by eating low-salt snacks. Remember salt, taken in the right amount is good for you. Teach yourself more about salt. Read the nutritional charts of your snacks.

Another way to watch your salt intake is to use seasonings with no salt. Other seasonings you can use in place of salt are cumin, black pepper, oregano, and many more. Alternatively, use seasoning sparingly so that you don't use too much.

And I can't forget about salty snacks. Those are the best snacks, but not very good for us. Substitute chips for fruits and unsalted nuts. Some grocery stores sell vegetable platters, make a habit of buying one, and use them for snacking.

In my opinion, if we reverse the way we have been living, our bodies will thank us by giving us fewer problems.

**Make a list of foods that you love with the most sodium, write them, and keep a diary of how often you are consuming them in the spaces provided. Make a daily effort to cut down the sodium intake.**

For example, I ate three bags of chips this week. The following week reduce by one bag until you can achieve to spend a week without chips. Replace them with healthy nuts.

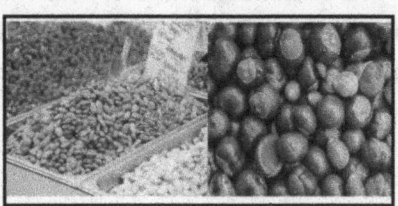

USING THE SPACES PROVIDED, write down a list of foods that are high in salts and make an effort to reduce the amount of sodium intake in your diary. All the best!

. . .

_____

_____

_____

_____

_____

# 7
## FATS

---

Alright, let's talk about the thing that people think they should avoid in their diet: fats. While most people are trying to lose weight, the one thing they want to avoid is the "F" word. But there is nothing wrong with having fats in your diet, as long as it benefits you. Let's talk about this in-depth.

Fats are important as part of a healthy diet. They provide essential fatty acids and give us energy. There are two types of fat: good and bad. To have a balanced diet, we need to learn the basics of good fats and bad fats. And yes, there are some fatty foods that are actually good for us.

Now, eating the right fatty foods is the hard part. Why? Because bad fatty foods are more appealing. The bad fatty foods are usually in the foods that most people eat often. The foods we love that have been ready-made are usually cooked in high fats, for example, good old fries. The frozen fries are less work and more attractive than peeling potatoes and making fresh ones. So, guess which one the busy working mom will purchase - yep, the frozen fries aka bad fatty food.

Like with anything else, when it comes to eating specific foods, moderation plays an important role. Healthy or not, too much fat in our diets causes obesity and illnesses like heart disease, and also research has shown that it can also trigger type 2 diabetes.

So, why should we add fats to our diets? They say we need small amounts of fat in our diets for healthy living. The oils and fats supply our bodies with calories, and essential fats that help our bodies absorb fat-soluble vitamins like A, D, E, and K.

The type of fat is just as important for health as the total amount of fat consumed. That's why it's important to choose healthier unsaturated fats. Eating too much and the wrong kinds of fats, such as saturated and trans fats, may raise unhealthy LDL cholesterol and lower healthy HDL cholesterol. This imbalance can increase risks of high blood pressure, hardening of the arteries (atherosclerosis), heart attack and stroke. Let's talk about the different types of fats.

**Monounsaturated Fats** have been shown to improve blood cholesterol levels. They are found in one of the following. They contain nine calories of fat per gram.

- Olive oil - which comes from olives and the oil is made by pressing the olives.
- Canola oil- is a vegetable oil derived from a variety of rapeseed
- Peanut oil also known as groundnut oil, it is derived from peanuts
- Avocado is plant-based and belongs to the fruit's category
- Nuts such as hazelnuts, almonds, pistachios, pecans, and cashew

POLYUNSATURATED FATS also contain nine calories per gram. They contain fats that help bad cholesterol levels in a person's blood and lowers the risk of heart disease and stroke. Polyunsaturated fats are plant-based, and some examples are corn oil, sunflower oil, and soybean oil.

Omega-3 is a polyunsaturated fat, which helps prevent clotting blood, reduces the risk of stroke, and also helps lower triglycerides, a type of blood fat linked to heart disease. Omega-3 fats are mainly found in cold-water fish (mackerel, sardines, herring, rainbow trout, and salmon). Polyunsaturated fats also help reduce bad cholesterol levels in our blood, which can lower one's risk of heart disease and stroke. They provide nutrients to help develop and maintain healthy body's cells

- Canola and soybean oils
- Omega-3 eggs
- Flaxseed
- Walnuts
- Pecans and pine nuts

Another type of polyunsaturated fat is omega 6. It helps lower LDL cholesterol, but in large amounts, it's thought to also lower the good HDL cholesterol. Eat it in moderation. Omega-6 is found in safflower, sunflower and corn oils, non-hydrogenated margarine, and nuts, such as almonds, pecans, brazil nuts and sunflower seeds. It is also in many prepared meals.

SATURATED **Fats** raise bad (LDL) cholesterol. LDL cholesterol is a risk factor for heart disease and stroke. The goods that we love and are our everyday foods are unfortunately high in saturated fat. These foods are:

- Fatty meats
- Full-fat dairy products
- Butter
- Hard margarine
- Lard
- Coconut oil
- Ghee (clarified butter)
- Vegetable ghee

In Canada, highly and ultra-processed foods are our major source of saturated fats in our diets. Foods that are manufactured in processing plants sometimes go through a lot of changes and additives, so it tends to lose its nutritional value vs. the food that comes from farm to table. A few summers ago, I worked in a hot dog processing facility and unfortunately lost my appetite for hotdogs. An example of highly processed foods is hot dogs, hamburgers, French fries, and many more.

### Trans Fat

BEFORE I END THIS BOOK, I want to talk about Trans Fat. It's by far the most unhealthy fat. Medicine.net describes trans-fat as a substance that is made through the chemical process of hydrogenation of oils. Hydrogenation solidifies liquid oils and increases the shelf life and the flavor stability of oils and foods that contain them. Trans fats are the worst and very dangerous for us to consume.

I want to give a huge thank you to the Canadian government for banning the addition of trans fats to food products since September 2018. This is huge and I hope other countries follow suit. I also want to thank the Heart and Stroke foundation for playing an effective role in doing research and advocating for changes to the food.

Overindulging in foods that included trans-fat caused a huge bump in the road for my health. A few years ago after giving birth to my daughter, I went to the emergency room feeling like I was having a heart attack. I told the doctor what my symptoms were, and his response was, Do you have a family history of gallstones?

I said to him in Africa I have never heard of gallstones but gold stones (my sense of humor lol). Gallstones are a small, hard crystalline mass formed abnormally in the gallbladder or bile ducts from bile pigments, cholesterol, and calcium salts. These are not good. According to Mayoclinic.org, A gallstone can cause a blockage in the pancreatic duct, which can lead to inflammation of the pancreas (pancreatitis). Pancreatitis causes intense, constant abdominal pain and usually requires hospitalization.

While I may joke about having this in my bloodline or not, it's a very serious medical issue. Apparently, there were concerns about me having gallstones. I then went for an ultrasound and yes, they found the little devils in there. I cried my eyes out, and I then started thinking that I'd have to have surgery immediately. I got better and I started lots of research on how to live with gallstones and I googled everything under the sun to make sure that I never ever suffer another attack. To this day I haven't had another episode, and my daughter is now eight years old. I watch what I eat.

## Better Eating Habits

TO THIS DAY, as I write, I thank the Lord that I haven't. I did a lot of research and learned more about healthy fats and unhealthy fats.

In my experience, this has caused the gallbladder to function better without me feeling sick all the time. I reduced the amount of bad fats for good fats. I don't use any oil when I am cooking because I find that they have their own fats. I grill and bake my food instead of frying. I use coconut oil (sparingly), olive oil, and canola for other uses in the kitchen. Here is an example of how I cook chicken leg quarters.

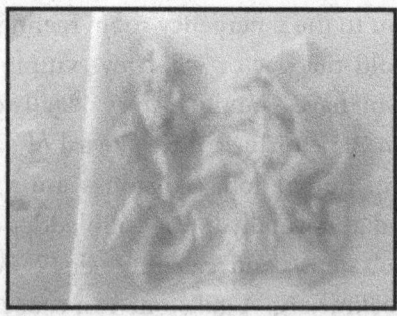

STEP 1 - REMOVE the skin

STEP 2 - USE chicken quarters with minimal fat. Now season the chicken with your favorite spices and also watch the salt quantity in some spices.

STEP 3 After seasoning your chicken, grill it on high in the oven and turn it roughly every 6 mins. After it has browned, I then baste it with salad dressing below. This makes your chicken moist, and you will end up with the finished chicken looking like the one in the picture below. Try it, and if you love the taste, kindly drop us a line at debunkdevelop@gmail.com with your testimonials. You will realize that the amount of bad fats you consume will decrease to a minimum as we replace them with good fats. Remember to do everything in moderation, personally, the small changes in my diet have kept my gallbladder at bay.

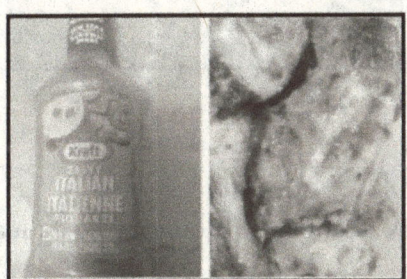

**Signature Scones**

ONE OF THE foods that I keep in my diet is scones and muffins. Luckily, I found a healthy way to eat them. I bake scones using coconut oil, and when making muffins I substitute butter with olive oil when baking muffins, and bread. The scones in the picture on the following page are good for school lunches, corporate meetings, parties, and many more.

Although coconut oil and butter are considered bad, just remember it's about the quantity of the fats we are consuming. Like everything in a diet, use them in moderation.

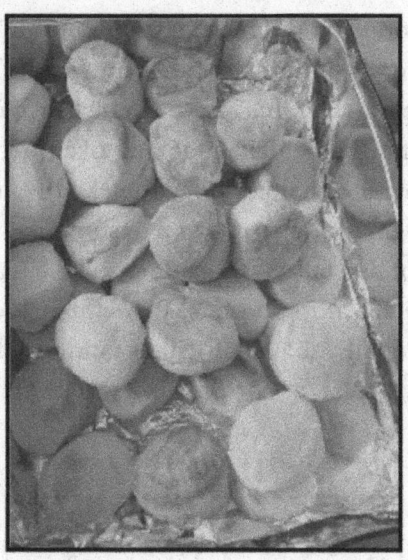

### How to Eat Fresh Home Cooked Meals

As a working parent who has three little kids, I understand how tiring cooking can be. I come home every day, like everyone else *tired*. Rather than cook daily, I decided to plan out our weekly meals. I pre-plan my meals for the week so that I spend less time in the kitchen. I recommend you set aside two hours of your time each day off and make ready-to-eat foods. Having cooked foods in the fridge and freezer will help you minimize that trip to a fast food joint as often.

Another way I eat home-cooked meals is that I make salads and cook beef in advance. You can also find recipes on Pinterest and allrecipes.com for ideas of how to cook anything you want. Happy clean eating!

## 8
# VITAMINS

---

I n order to live a healthy life, one must develop healthy eating habits. Here is an A-Z of essential foods and nutrients we must eat regularly to maintain good health.

INSTEAD OF CONSUMING daily doses of multivitamins, if our eating habits contain foods that have all the groups of vitamins we take in the form of pills, then we will be saving money. Instead of buying food plus vitamins, you will have one less thing to spend money on. Here is an example of vitamin-rich foods.

**Vitamin A**

VITAMIN A IS FOUND in leafy green foods like spinach, kale, and collard greens. Other Vitamin A foods are carrots, lettuce, pumpkin, squash, turnips, chard, apricots, asparagus, peas, and many more. I understand some people might not like some foods, but there are so many choices in every food group. Fall in love with a few and include them in your weekly seven-day eating habits.

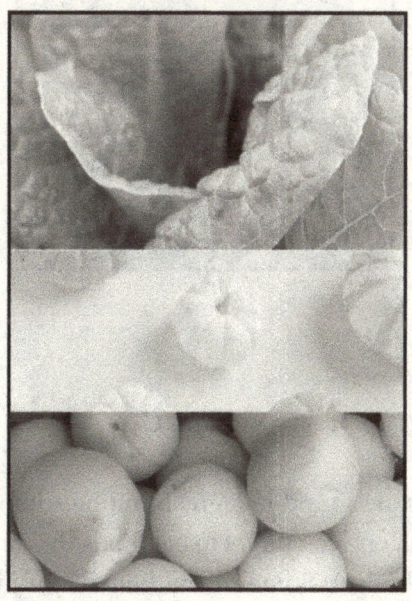

**Vitamin B**

The B vitamins are the G8 of powerful nutrients. They are a superpower of 8 nutrients, which are known as B1( thiamin), B2 (riboflavin) B3 (niacin) B5 (pantothenic acid) B6(pyridoxine) B7(biotin) B9 (folate is commonly known as folic acid) and B12 (cobalamin). It is recommended you eat a balanced diet in order to have adequate nutrients in your bodies. A balanced diet consists of meats, fish, bread, cereals, rice, fruit, and vegetables.

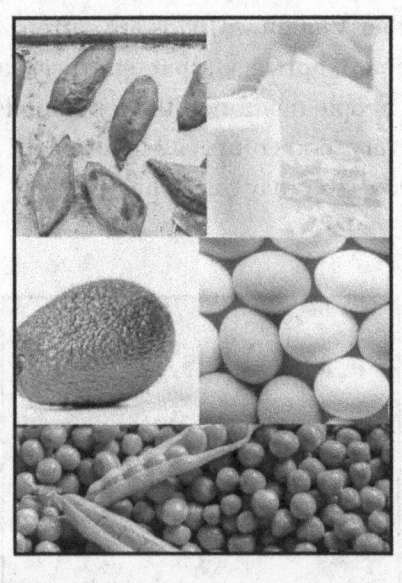

## Vitamin C

Vitamin C foods are found in a great number of foods. With a good daily food journal, one can target to eat foods that are high in vitamin C at a very low budget. Some of the benefits of vitamin C include immune system boosting, and helps protect your heart against diseases. Some of our favorite fruits are filled with vitamin C.

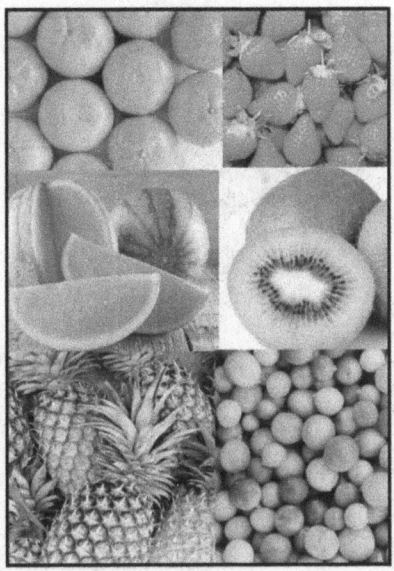

**Vitamin D**

Vitamin D is not found in many foods, but there are still great foods in its category. It is a nutrient that a person's skin absorbs when they are in direct sunlight. It's mainly from the sun as we read earlier in sun facts. Vitamin D is also found in fortified foods like oatmeal, fortified cereals, and milk. Because of winter, where we have limited time, it's recommended to use Vitamin D supplements daily.

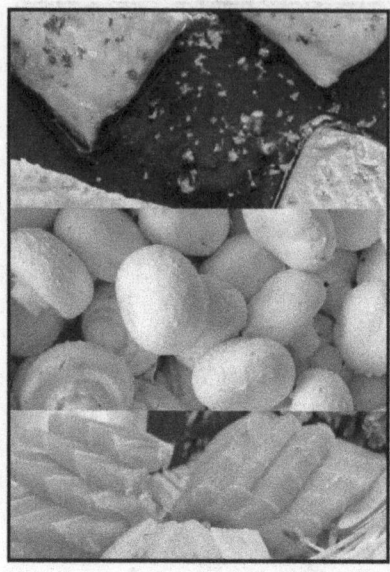

## Vitamin E

A LOT of fruits and vegetables are like multi-level marketing. They are interconnected with great benefits with the common goal of making it to the top. The more you invest in healthy eating, the longer you live and reap the benefits. Vitamin E is also found in oils. It is essential for skin moisturizing and is also known for its antioxidants, which the body utilizes to protect our skin and repair cells.

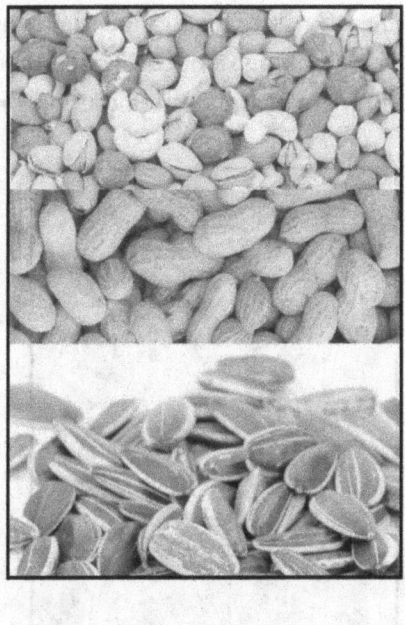

## Fish Oil

Fish oils are known to reduce heart disease and some cancers, according to research. It's known to help lower blood pressure during pregnancy. Having been pregnant and experienced the different stages of love and hate relationship with food, in this case, I recommend taking multivitamins. Fish oils can be found on foods on the vitamin D chart, which are, Salmon, mushrooms, and tuna. I advise using caution with tuna while pregnant. I also recommend you talk to your doctor.

## Magnesium

AS I MENTIONED EARLIER, most foods are part of a pyramid. Their networks and net worth are somewhat linked. Magnesium is found in leafy vegetables—avocados, banana, and foods that contain fiber. If you are following the A-Z of the food guide, then you are getting this nutrient without even thinking about it. Foods that contain various amounts of magnesium are peanut butter, quinoa, bran, and corn.

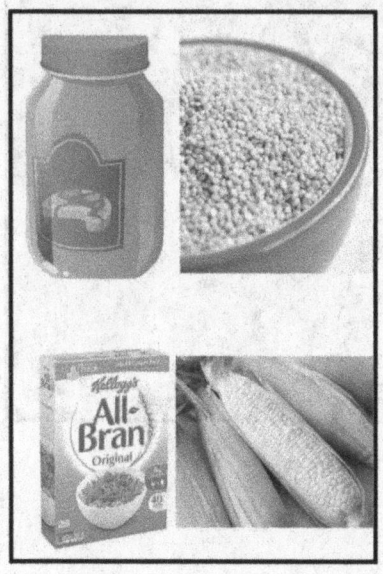

### Potassium

In the right amounts, potassium is an essential service of our bodies. We need it in order to have our cells function in a healthy way. Some people who have potassium deficiency will experience muscle cramps, numbing and other symptoms. Always seek professional help and never self-diagnose. Here are foods that have potassium in them.

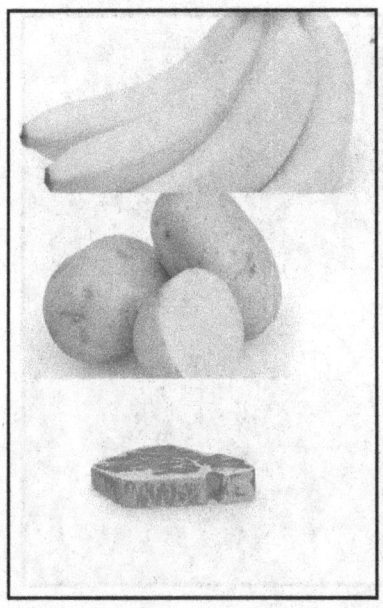

## Zinc

Our bodies require this precious mineral, just like gold is a unique mineral in the world of minerals. The body only requires a trace amount of zinc. It's found in meats, dairy and aids in wound healing and, above all, a healthy immune function.

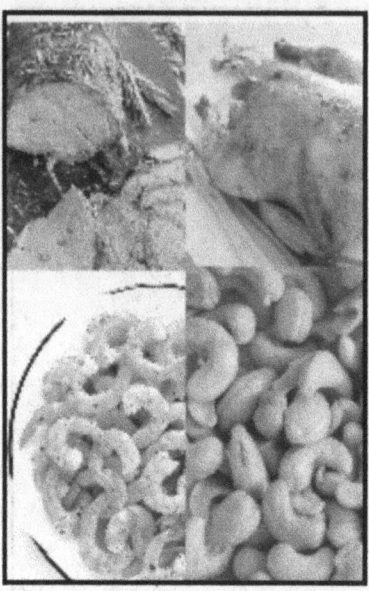

The food groups gathered here are just for guidance. Many nutritious foods belong to the same food groups and complement each other by providing different nutrients in our bodies.

As mentioned earlier, other vitamins like Vitamin K are interlinked to the food pyramid and also found in fats, calcium is found in milk, iron is found in meats, nuts, and whole grains. Another vitamin is Selenium, which is found in brazil nuts. The secret to living a healthy life starts with you by implementing life changes. Happy Reversing!

In order to live a reversed lifestyle, one must include daily activities in their routine. Here is an A-Z list of activities you can incorporate into your life as part of a healthy living routine.

- Aerobics.
- Biking, bowling, bocce, burpees, bicycle
- Cycling, crunch
- Dancing's, dumbbells, donkey kicks
- Elliptical
- Football, frisbee

- Golf, Gymnastics
- Hiking
- Interval training
- Jogging, jumping jacks
- Kickboxing, Kettlebell
- Lightweights, lunges
- Move any movement
- Netball
- Oblique hanging leg raise
- Pilates, pushup , planks
- Quadriceps
- Running,
- Swimming, skipping rope, soccer, squats, single-leg deadlifts, sit-ups, side planks, step up
- Tennis. Tai Chi
- Use your imagination to think of an exercise and create your own
- Walking
- Exhale in and out. Breathe in and out
- Yoga
- Zumba

I HOPE READING this book has opened your eyes and nudged you to start living a reversed life. While I understand that our lives are hectic work, home, and extracurricular activities, just doing small changes like cooking a couple of meals in advance will help you eat more made at home goods and made at home is cheaper than takeaway. There is a saying that saying a little goes a long way and 500 million people made small changes that will improve our lives and reduce wasting energy and lessening our dump yards with excessive waste. I would love to hear your feedback about what you learned and how it resonates with you. Please drop me an email at debunkdevelop@gmail.com

. . .

READY, Set, Go, and Live your life in Reverse. Change begins with You!!

*Resources*

I WOULD LOVE to thank the following organizations who made it possible for me to add previous research to support LYLIR on health topics.

- Mayoclinic.org
- Wikipedia
- Encyclopedia Britannica
- Canada.ca
- Desygner
- NBCnews.com

## WHO IS LUCY RUTH?

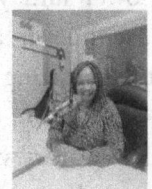

Lucy is an author and a public speaker. She is a Guinness World Record Holder (The Most Authors Signing The Same Book at The Same Time). Her first book titled "Debunk & Develop Your Mind" was published on March 28, 2019, and became a #1 bestseller on Amazon. Her second book was titled "How to Love Yourself after Bullying and Abuse."

Her efforts to inspire those in her community and abroad have led to networking opportunities with many public figures who have endorsed her work. She is a mother of three, works full time, and also runs an online business selling African heritage products on Amazon. In 2018, Lucy was featured in a story by The Weight She Carries for her support of African artistry. The trajectory of her life changed at the age of ten when she lost her mother in her native, Zimbabwe. For years, Lucy struggled with depression and felt alone because depression was not a topic people discussed in Zimbabwe. This birthed a desire to connect with people.

Having lived and worked in three continents: Africa, Europe, and now North America, Lucy has been exposed to different cultures and experiences. While customs vary, she has seen a common thread in every place she has lived; the challenges people face are the same.

Gifted in being a good listener, Lucy is the voice of those who cannot stand up for themselves. She is passionate about equal opportunities for all and the empowerment of all people. Lucy has an ongoing relationship with the prison and is working on creating a self-help course for women who have served their time to rise and become tomorrow's leaders, Lucy manages and moderates a growing group for Strong Women on Facebook, which has 425 000 women worldwide. Lucy has the vision to empower and young men and women to believe in themselves and chase their dreams. Lucy is also part of the Toronto Women's Expo 2020 organizing committee. The expo and charity Gala in partnership with Million-dollar smiles charity, which builds playgrounds for sick kids countrywide.

Some of her notable accomplishments include:

- *Keynote Speaker for the Well and Black History Month 2019*
- *Keynote Speaker for Mother's Day at K.I.M Toronto*
- *Speaker at Grand Valley Women's Prison*
- *Speaker at Women's Economic Forum London 2019*
- *Speaker at Edo Women Conference Jan 2020*
- *Guest on Nebo TV speaking on mental health*
- *Guest on Aris eF.M. (Christian Radio)*
- *Award Nominee for Women making an impact Egypt March 2020*
- *Remarkable Mother's Day award upcoming in May 2020*
- *Guest on Radio Ink live with Kelly B. Hunter*

IN ADDITION, Lucy has experience in airport operations and was an airport Supervisor at London Gatwick airport. She has an education in airline and travel and is a holder of 30 IATA points. She also has an education in events management with public relations.

CONTACT: info@lucyruth.page

Website: www.lucyruth.page

FOLLOW LUCY:
   Linkedin: linkedin.com/in/lucy-r-b546b113
   Official website: https://www.lucyruth.page/
   Email: info@lucyruth.page

www.ingramcontent.com/pod-product-compliance
Lightning Source LLC
Chambersburg PA
CBHW010028040426
42333CB00047B/2722